Buttercre&

Tip 1: Do now no longer overbeat your b   ~eating butter
with none additives, which include sugar, :   , ~eat butter so long as you
desire.

Butter is available in extraordinary colors: pale, yellow, or orange. Typically,
you'll beat the butter for one to 2 mins, however If you need to gain a lighter
buttercream color, beat butter for an extended time.

Tip 2: Once you brought another elements to the butter, restrict beating to
twenty to 30 seconds or less.

Tip 3: Sift powdered sugar as a minimum one time to save you the advent of
lumps and creating a smoother buttercream.

Tip 4: When you're beating buttercream, make certain you periodically
scrape the edges of the bowl and mixer blades to comprise and calmly blend
all elements.

Tip five: Use cane sugar in place of beet sugar to gain a smoother
consistency.

Tip 6: If your buttercream is just too stiff, upload water or milk, one spoon at a
time.

Tip 7: If you need to apply buttercream for piping decorations, location it
withinside the refrigerator to chill earlier than the usage of.

Butter

Buttercream Ingredients

Buttercream recipes name for softened butter. What does this mean? Softened
butter need to maintain form whilst pressed down through a finger. Typically,
relying at the temperature to your kitchen, it takes among thirty mins to an
hour to melt the butter. You can accelerate the system through unwrapping
and reducing the butter into pieces.

Sugar

Depending at the recipe, you'll use both powdered sugar or granulated sugar.
Granulated sugar is utilized in meringue-primarily based totally buttercream
recipes. These recipes require heating, and granulated sugar melts properly
whilst it's far heated.

Powdered sugar is utilized in recipes that don't incorporate eggs. Powdered sugar combined with butter creates a easy consistency.

You need to sift powdered sugar earlier than blending it with butter to save you from developing lumps to your buttercream.

Do now no longer use granulated sugar in non-meringue buttercream due to the fact you'll sense sugar granules withinside the recipe.

It is pleasant to apply cane sugar (now no longer beet sugar) to create the pleasant texture and fine of buttercream.

Eggs

Some buttercream recipes name for the usage of eggs whilst others do now no longer require eggs. Meringue-primarily based totally buttercreams make it less difficult to pipe complicated shapes.

There is a way, however, to make eggless buttercream extra solid and applicable for piping. When you upload cornstarch or corn flour, your buttercream will become extra solid.

Make certain to apply natural corn starch and corn flour as corn merchandise are possibly to be genetically manipulated (GMO).

You can pasteurize uncooked eggs earlier than you upload them to a recipe.

To pasteurize eggs, location a water-proof bowl right into a saucepan. Add water to cowl 1/2 of of the bowl's height.

Place eggs into the bowl and warmth the water as much as 140°F. Let the water boil for approximately 3 mins to warmth up the eggs. Do now no longer permit the water warmth over

142°F.

Milk & Heavy Cream

When you're including milk to buttercream, make certain it's far entire milk. Whole milk includes a bigger quantity of fat. Alternatively, in place of including milk, you may upload heavy cream.

Vanilla Extract

Vanilla complements flavors. For instance, if the recipe makes use of chocolate, coffee, or fruit syrups, including vanilla complements the taste of additives.

Vanilla extract is available in herbal and synthetic forms. A herbal vanilla extract is advanced to synthetic vanilla extract. To create the pleasant fine buttercream, use herbal vanilla extract.

Almond Extract

The primary buttercream recipe does now no longer name for the usage of almond extract. Almond extract, however, complements the taste.

Pure almond extract consists of 3 number one elements: alcohol, water, and almond oil. To create the pleasant fine buttercream and to feature extra richness on your buttercream, use herbal almond extract.

Other ingredients

There are different elements that you may upload to the buttercream. This consists of fruit jellies, nuts, sparkling fruits, nut butter, and extra.

Recipes

1. Lavender and Vanilla Buttercream Frosting

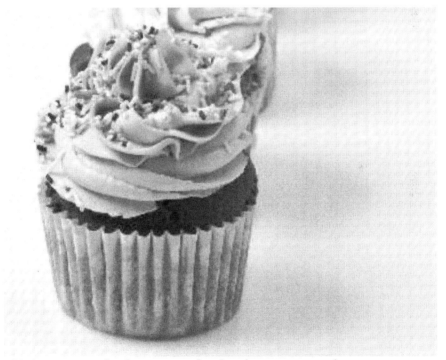

This is a great-tasting buttercream frosting that you may make on every occasion you're in want of a late-night time snack.

Serving Size: 4 servings

Cooking Time: 10 minutes

Ingredient:

- 1 cup of butter, soft

- 4 cups of powdered sugar
- 2 teaspoons of lavender extract
- 1 drop of purple food coloring

Instructions:

In a massive bowl, upload withinside the gentle butter. Beat with an electric powered mixer for 2

mins or till easy consistency.

Add withinside the lavender extract and red meals coloring. Continue to overcome for a further minute.

Gently upload withinside the powdered sugar and maintain to overcome for five mins or till fluffy consistency.

Use immediately.

2. Orange Cream Cheese Buttercream

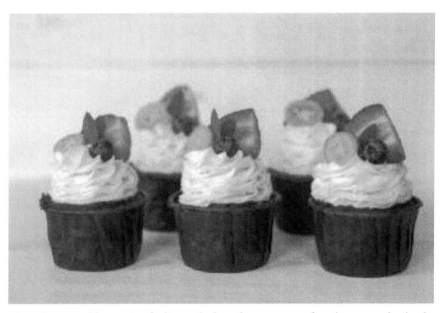

If you're searching out a fruity and clean buttercream frosting to make in the course of the summer time season months, then that is one buttercream recipe you may need to have for your arsenal.

Serving Size: 8 servings

Cooking Time: 25 minutes

Ingredient:

- 1 cup of unsalted butter, soft
- 4 ounces of cream cheese, chilled
- ½ cup of prepared orange curd
- 1 tablespoon of orange zest, grated
- ¼ teaspoon of Sicilia extract
- 4 to 4 ½ cups of powdered sugar
- 1 to 2 drops of orange food coloring

Instructions:

In the big bowl of a stand mixer, upload withinside the butter. Beat on the bottom placing to a creamy consistency.

Add withinside the cream cheese, orange curd, clean orange zest, and Sicilia extract. Beat till calmly incorporated.

Add withinside the powdered sugar and hold to overcome till clean consistency.

Add withinside the orange meals coloring and beat for an extra minute till mixed.

Increase the rate to medium and beat for five mins or till fluffy consistency.

Use right now.

3. Swiss Meringue Buttercream

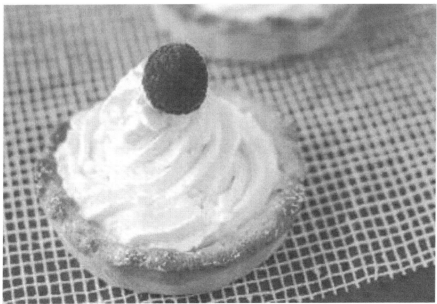

This is possibly one of the simplest meringue buttercream frosting recipes you may ever find. One taste, and you may placed it on almost everything.

Serving Size: 8 servings

Cooking Time: 12 minutes

Ingredient:

- ¾ cup of egg whites
- 6 cups of powdered sugar
- ½ teaspoon pf salt
- 3 cups of unsalted butter
- 2 tablespoons of pure vanilla

Instructions:

In the big bowl of a stand mixer, upload withinside the egg whites, powdered sugar, and sprint of salt.

Beat collectively on the bottom placing or till moist.

Increase the rate to medium and slowly upload withinside the unsalted butter. Continue to overcome.

Add withinside the natural vanilla.

Beat on the bottom placing for 10 mins or till creamy consistency. Use right now or shop withinside the refrigerator to chill.

4. Bailey's Buttercream

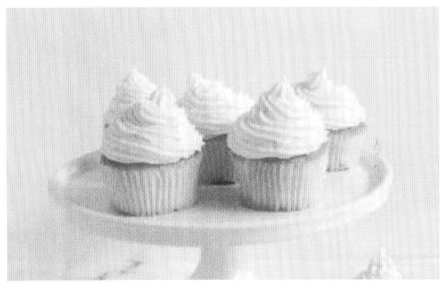

If you need to make adult-pleasant cupcakes or cake, then that is the appropriate buttercream to pair together with them.

Serving Size: 12 servings

Cooking Time: 10 minutes

Ingredients:

- 1 cup of butter, cut into small cubes
- 2 ¼ cups of powdered sugar
- 2 ½ tablespoons of Bailey's Irish Cream

Instructions:

Add the butter cubes right into a big bowl. Beat with an electric powered mixer till creamy consistency.

Gently upload withinside the powdered sugar and hold to overcome till creamy. Add withinside the Bailey's slowly. Beat to mix.

Continue to overcome for five mins or till fluffy in consistency. Use right now.

5. Vegan Buttercream Frosting

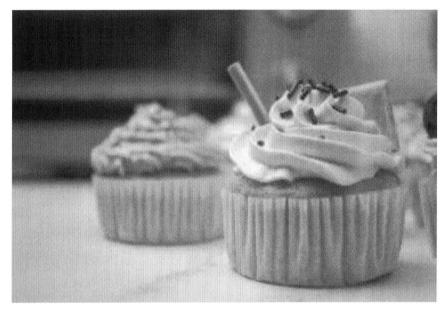

This is the appropriate frosting to make to your vegan buddies and family. It pairs excellently with vegan pleasant cake or cupcakes.

Serving Size: 6 servings

Cooking Time: 20 minutes

Ingredients:

- 1 cup of powdered sugar
- 1 cup of vegetable shortening
- 2 drops of pure vanilla
- 1 tablespoon of almond milk
- 2 drops of pink food coloring

Instructions:

In a big bowl, upload withinside the vegetable shortening. Beat with an electric powered mixer on the bottom placing for 7 to eight mins or till clean consistency.

Add withinside the natural vanilla and mix once more till calmly incorporated.

Add withinside the powdered sugar, almond milk and purple meals coloring. Blend at the medium placing till calmly mixed.

Continue to overcome for five to 7 mins or till fluffy

consistency. Use right now.

6. Salted Caramel Buttercream Frosting

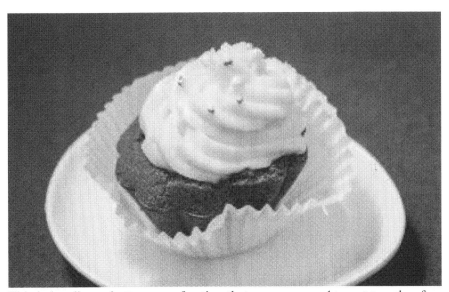

This is handiest a buttercream frosting that you may need to put together for the greatest of occasions. It takes a chunk extra attempt than maximum buttercream frostings, however it's miles nicely really well worth the attempt withinside the end.

Serving Size: 24 servings

Cooking Time: 10 minutes

Ingredients:

- 1 cup of butter, soft
- 1/3 cup of salted caramel sauce
- 1 teaspoon of pure vanilla
- 1 ½ cups of powdered sugar
- Dash of salt

Instructions:

In a big bowl, upload withinside the gentle butter. Beat with an electric powered mixer till clean consistency.

Add withinside the caramel sauce and natural vanilla. Continue to overcome for two mins or till clean.

Add withinside the sprint of salt and powdered sugar. Beat on the bottom placing for two mins or till calmly incorporated.

Increase the rate of the mixer to medium. Continue to overcome for two to a few mins or till fluffy consistency.

Use right now.

7. Double Chocolate Buttercream

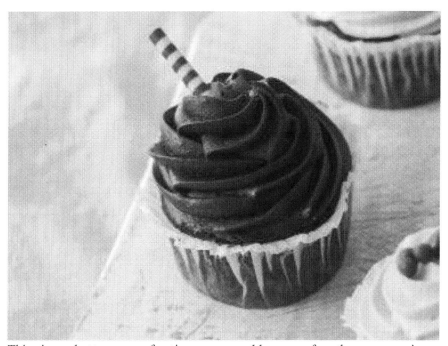

This is a buttercream frosting you could serve for the ones unique chocoholics for your home. It is so tasty, even the pickiest eaters will fall in love with it.

Serving Size: 2 ½ servings

Cooking Time: 5 minutes

Ingredients:

- 1 cup of unsalted butter, soft
- 3 ½ cups of powdered sugar
- ½ cup of powdered unsweetened cocoa
- 3 tablespoons of heavy cream

- ¼ teaspoon of salt
- 2 teaspoons of pure vanilla

Instructions:

n the big bowl of a stand mixer, upload withinside the unsalted butter. Beat on the very best placing till creamy consistency.

Add withinside the powdered sugar, powdered cocoa, heavy cream, sprint of salt and natural vanilla.

Reduce the rate to low and hold to overcome for three mins or till fluffy consistency.

Use right now or shop withinside the refrigerator to chill.

8. White Chocolate Buttercream

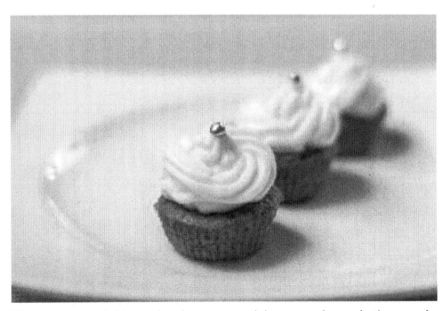

This is a remarkable tasting buttercream icing to make each time you're yearning chocolate or white chocolate. Decadent in taste, that is the appropriate frosting to apply for layer cakes.

Serving Size: 12 servings

Cooking Time: 10 minutes

Ingredients:

- 1 cup of unsalted butter, soft
-

1 cup of powdered sugar
- ¾ cup of white chocolate
- Splash of whole milk

Instructions:

Break the white chocolate into small pieces. Place right into a small bowl. Microwave for 30 seconds or till melted.

In the big bowl of a stand mixer, upload withinside the unsalted butter.

Beat collectively on the very best placing till creamy consistency.

Add withinside the melted white chocolate, powdered sugar and splash of complete milk. Continue to overcome for eight mins or till fluffy consistency.

Use right now or shop withinside the refrigerator to chill.

9. Brown Sugar Buttercream

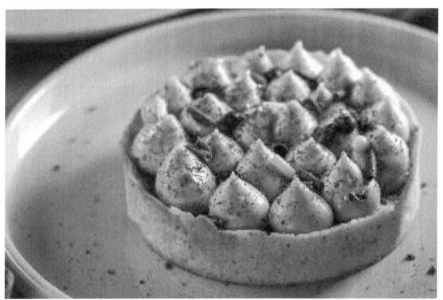

This is a buttercream frosting this is much like the Swiss meringue frosting, simply a chunk sweeter. It is best for almost any cake that you can make.

Serving Size: 4 servings

Cooking Time: 10 minutes

Ingredients:

- 6 egg whites

- 1 2/3 cups of light brown sugar
- ¼ teaspoon of salt
- 4 sticks of unsalted butter, soft

Instructions:

In a big bowl, upload withinside the egg whites and mild brown sugar. Place the bowl over a pot that consists of 1 inch of boiling water. Stir nicely till the sugar is absolutely melted.

Remove from the pot. Beat the sugar with an electric powered mixer at the medium

placing till stiff consistency.

Add withinside the gentle butter and sprint of salt. Continue to overcome for five mins or till glossy.

Use at once.

10. Chocolate Mousse Buttercream Frosting

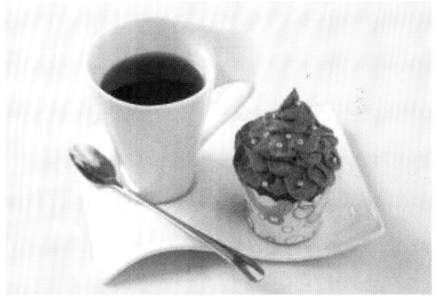

If you're searching out the precise buttercream frosting to make to destroy your pals and family, then that is the precise frosting with the intention to make.

Serving Size: 6 servings

Cooking Time: 30 minutes

Ingredients:

- 10 ounces of milk chocolate, chopped
- 6 ounces of dark chocolate, chopped
- 1 ½ cups of heavy whipping cream
- 2 tablespoons of golden syrup
- 1 cup of salted butter, soft
- ¾ cup of unsalted butter, soft

Instructions:

In a big bowl, upload withinside the chopped milk and darkish chocolate. Stir properly to combine. Place a small saucepan over medium warmness. Add withinside the heavy whipping cream

and golden syrup. Whisk to combine and produce to a boil. Immediately dispose of from warmness and pour the cream aggregate over the chocolate. Stir properly till the chocolate melts.

Add withinside the gentle salted and unsalted butter. Beat on the bottom putting for six to eight mins or till fluffy consistency.

Transfer into the freezer to relax for five mins earlier than the use of.

11. Guinness Buttercream

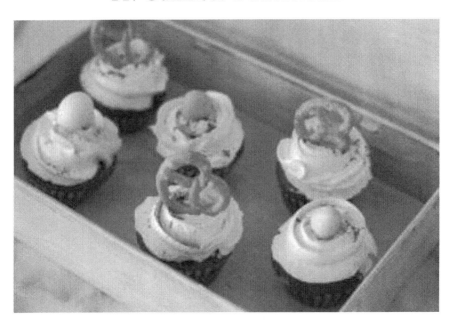

A wealthy beer is going wonderful in buttercream. Cooking the beer earlier than the use of it allows you to get extra taste packed into the frosting and additionally makes this buttercream nonalcoholic.

Serving Size: Frosting for 24 cupcakes

Cooking Time: 35 Minutes

Ingredients:

- 1 cup Guinness beer
- 1 cup Butter
- 3 cups powdered sugar
- 1 teaspoon vanilla
- 1/2 teaspoon Salt

Instructions:

In a small saucepan, deliver 1 cup of Guinness boil. Turn down the warmth to medium-low and allow simmer till the combinationture has decreased via way of means of 1/2 of and is a thick

syrup for approximately 15-20 mins.

Remove from warmness and set apart to cool.

In a mixer with a paddle attachment, cream the butter and powdered sugar till tremendous fluffy and light; the combinationture have to flip white; take into account to scrape down the bowl numerous times.

Add the salt, vanilla, and Guinness syrup and beat again, scraping down the bowl to comprise everything. Use at once or keep at room temp for up to three days.

12. Cannoli Cream Buttercream

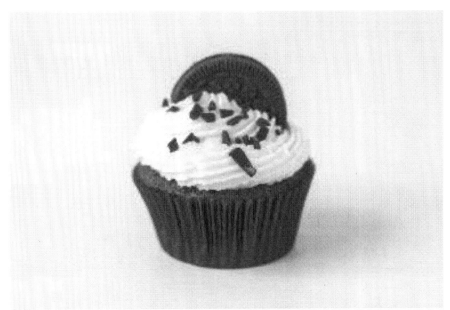

If you adore cannoli cake or normal cannolis, then you definitely should do that recipe! A move among cannoli filling and creamy buttercream, you simply can't pass incorrect right here!

Serving Size: Frosting for 36 cupcakes or one 8" Cake

Cooking Time: 35 minutes

Ingredients:

- 6 cups Sugar
- 1 3/4 cups egg whites
- 2 teaspoons Vanilla Extract
- 1/2 teaspoon Salt
- 2 1/2 cups Butter, softened
- 1 cup ricotta impastata
- 1 cup powdered sugar

Instructions:

Measure the sugar right into a big pot and cowl it with water. Stir so there's no dry sugar at the lowest of the pot.

Boil the sugar till it reaches 238 F on a sweet thermometer; do now no longer stir the sugar at the same time as it's far boiling as this can reason it to crystallize.

While you're looking forward to the sugar to boil, area the egg whites right into a mixer with a whisk attachment and whip to gentle peaks.

While the mixer is on, whipping the eggs, slowly upload the new sugar aggregate (slowly is prime right here so you do now no longer prepare dinner dinner the egg whites

After the sugar is added, preserve to whip the whites for approximately 20 mins or till the bowl is cool to the touch.

Slowly upload chunks of butter to the egg white mix, constantly with the mixer on, till all of the butter is in and the icing has come collectively to appearance thick and fluffy.

Add the ricotta impastata and powdered sugar and blend at low velocity till simply incorporated.

Add the vanilla and salt and use at once or keep withinside the refrigerator for up to 1 week.

13. Deluxe Cannoli Cream Buttercream

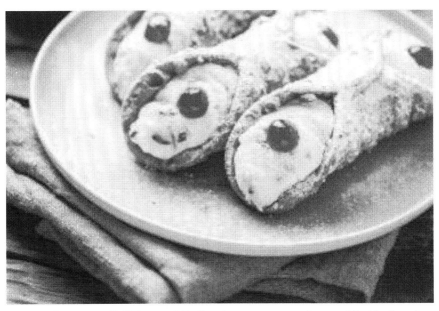

True Italian cannoli filling and Italian buttercream unite on this ideal recipe. Subtle notes of orange and lemon emphasize the cannoli flavor and chocolate chips (at the same time as optional) placed this frosting over the edge.

Serving Size: Frosting for 36 cupcakes or one 8" Cake

Cooking Time: 35 minutes

Ingredients:

- 6 cups Sugar
- 1 3/4 cups egg whites
- 2 teaspoons Vanilla Extract
- 1/2 teaspoon Salt
- 2 1/2 cups Butter, softened
- 1 cup ricotta impastata
- 1 cup powdered sugar
- 1 teaspoon orange zest
- 1/2 teaspoon lemon zest
- 1 cup mini chocolate chips (optional)

Instructions:

Measure the sugar right into a big pot and cowl it with water. Stir so there's no dry sugar at the lowest of the pot

Boil the sugar till it reaches 238 F on a sweet thermometer. Do now no longer stir the sugar at the same time as it's far boiling, as this can reason it to crystallize.

While you're looking forward to the sugar to boil, area the egg whites right into a mixer with a whisk attachment and whip to gentle peaks.

While the mixer is on, whipping the eggs, slowly upload the new sugar aggregate (slowly is prime right here so you do now no longer prepare dinner dinner the egg whites

After the sugar is added, preserve to whip the whites for approximately 20 mins or till the bowl is cool to the touch.

Slowly upload chunks of butter to the egg white mix, constantly with the mixer on, till all of the butter is in and the icing has come collectively to appearance thick and fluffy.

Add the ricotta impastata, orange zest, lemon zest, and powdered sugar and blend on low velocity till simply incorporated.

Fold withinside the mini chocolate chips via way of means of hand in case you are the use of them.

Add the vanilla and salt and use at once or keep withinside the refrigerator for up to 1 week.

14. Tiramisu Buttercream

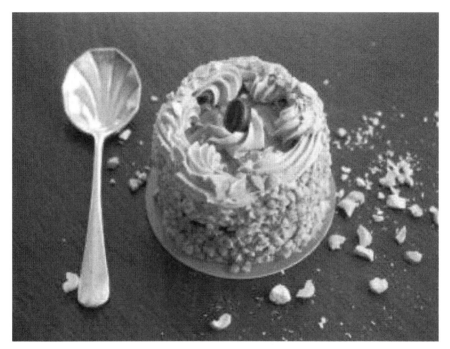

Using an Italian buttercream base, this recipe then provides rum, coffee, and mascarpone flavors to make this buttercream a dessert in itself. Use chocolate or vanilla desserts at the outside and inside for a really perfect dessert.

Serving Size: Frosting for 48 cupcakes or one 10" Cake

Cooking Time: 35 minutes

Ingredients:

- 6 cups Sugar
- 3/4 cup coffee
- 1 3/4 cups egg whites
- 1 teaspoon coffee extract
- 2 teaspoons Rum Extract
- 1/2 teaspoon Salt
- 2 1/2 cups Butter, softened
- 1 cup heavy cream
- 1 cup mascarpone cheese

Instructions:

Measure the sugar right into a big pot and upload coffee. Stir so there's no dry sugar at the lowest of the pot

Boil the sugar till it reaches 238 F on a sweet thermometer; do now no longer stir the sugar whilst it's miles boiling as this can reason it to crystallize.

While you're watching for the sugar to boil, vicinity the egg whites right into a mixer with a whisk attachment and whip to gentle peaks.

While the mixer is on, whipping the eggs, slowly upload the new sugar mixture (slowly is prime right here so you do now no longer prepare dinner dinner the egg whites

After the sugar is added, retain to whip the whites for approximately 20 mins or till the bowl is cool to the touch.

Slowly upload chunks of butter to the egg white blend, constantly with the mixer on, till all of the butter is in and the icing has come collectively to appearance thick and fluffy.

Add the rum extract, espresso extract, and salt. Set the buttercream apart

In a smooth bowl, whisk the heavy cream and mascarpone cheese collectively till stiff peaks form.

Fold the whipped cream and mascarpone blend into the organized buttercream and use straight away.

15. Coconut Cream Buttercream

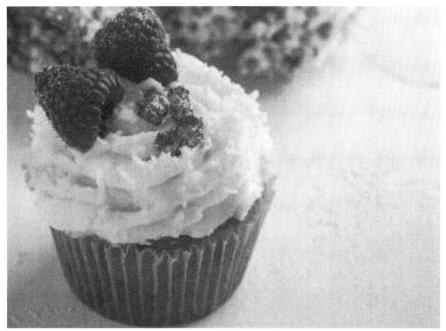

Made the usage of the German technique of creating buttercream, this recipe has you first make a pastry cream with coconut milk. The wealthy cream is then whipped collectively with butter for a wealthy and scrumptious frosting.

Serving Size: frosting for 36 cupcakes

Cooking Time: 30 minutes

Ingredients:

- 1 cup full fat coconut milk
- 1/8 cup sugar
- 2 eggs
- 1/8 cup corn starch
- 1/4 cup sugar
- 1 teaspoon Vanilla
- 2 pounds butter
- 1/2 cup powdered sugar
- 1/2 cup shredded coconut

Instructions:

In a medium bowl, whisk collectively the cornstarch and the 1/four cup sugar. Add the eggs final and whisk collectively.

In a small saucepan, deliver the coconut milk and 1/eight cup sugar to a boil. Pour the boiling milk into the cornstarch blend, whisking constantly.

Put the entirety again into the saucepan and prepare dinner dinner on low warmness, constantly
stirring till the combinationture has thickened. Remove from the warmth and upload the vanilla stress if any lumps have formed.

Place a chunk of plastic wrap immediately at the pinnacle of the pastry cream and vicinity it withinside the refrigerator to chill absolutely.

In the bowl of a stand mixer geared up with a paddle attachment, cream the powdered sugar and butter till very fluffy and light. Scrape down the edges of the bowl as needed

Add the cooled pastry cream into the butter approximately 1/four of a cup at a time. Mix properly in among every addition.

Once all of the cream has been added, use the buttercream straight away or shop it withinside the refrigerator for as much as a week.

.

16. Brownie Buttercream

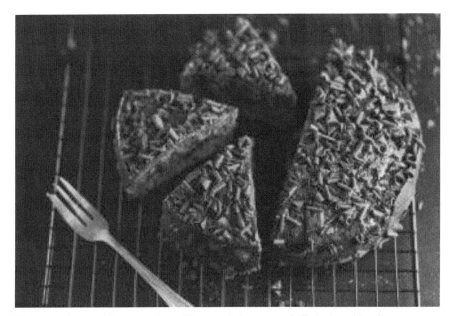

First, you're making actual truffles, and then you definitely whip them up

right into a cream cheese-primarily based totally buttercream for a frosting this is natural perfection.

Serving Size: 24

Cooking Time: 35 Minutes

Brownie Ingredients:

- 3 tablespoons Butter
- 1/4 cup Sugar
- 1 teaspoon Vanilla
- 3/4 cup mini semisweet chocolate chips
- 1 egg
- 1 tablespoon Dark Cocoa Powder
- 1/2 tablespoon Tapioca Flour
- 1/4 teaspoon Salt

Instructions:

In a small saucepan over low warmness, soften the butter.

Add the mini chocolate chips to the butter and stir to soften the chips. Remove from the warmth.

Add the vanilla and eggs to the chocolate to the saucepan and blend thoroughly. four. Sift tapioca and cocoa powder into the chocolate blend and stir

Add the salt to the chocolate and blend the entirety collectively.

Pour the truffles right into a properly-greased 8x8" rectangular pan (they may be thin) and right into a 350 F oven. Bake for 15 mins and get rid of from oven. Allow the truffles to chill withinside the pan after which cool absolutely withinside the refrigerator as they may be less complicated to reduce whilst very cold.

Brownie Buttercream Ingredients:

- 1 batch of brownies
- 1 pound butter
- 1/2 pound cream cheese
- 2 cups powdered sugar

Buttercream Instructions:

In a blending bowl with a paddle attachment, cream the cream cheese and butter collectively.

Add the powdered sugar and beat till very fluffy and light; the combinationture ought to be essentially white.

Add the truffles into the mixer in chunks and blend on medium velocity to mash them into the buttercream.

Scrape down the bowl often to make certain the entirety is combined. Mix till smooth, then use straight away.

17. Margarita Buttercream

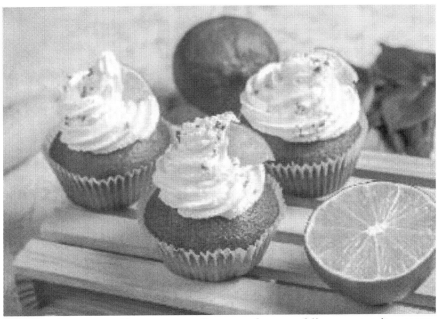

The cool summer time season flavors of a sparkling margarita cross flawlessly with this creamy buttercream. Try this with a lemon or lime cake and pair it with a few scrumptious lemon curd as properly.

Serving Size: Frosting for 24 cupcakes

Cooking Time: 35 Minutes

Ingredients:

- 1/2 cup tequila
- 1/8 cup sugar
- 1 cup Butter
- 3 cups powdered sugar
- 1 teaspoon Salt
- 2 teaspoons lime zest

Instructions:

In a small saucepan, deliver the tequila and sugar to a boil. Turn the warmth right all the way down to medium-low and allow simmer till the combinationture has decreased via way of means of 1/2 of and is a thick syrup for approximately 15-20 mins.

Remove from warmness after which set apart to chill.

In a mixer with a paddle attachment, cream the butter and powdered sugar till terrific fluffy and light; the combinationture ought to flip white; recollect to scrape down the bowl numerous times.

Add the salt, tequila, and lime zest and beat again, scraping down the bowl to include the entirety. Use straight away or shop at room temp for up to three days.

18. Dulce de Leche Buttercream

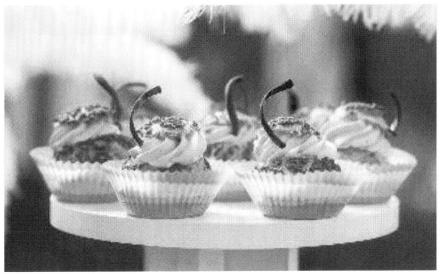

This is a buttercream recipe loaded with a ton of caramel flavor, making it best for making vanilla or chocolate cakes.

Serving Size: 36 servings

Cooking Time: 35 minutes

Ingredients:

- 6 cups of white sugar
- 1 ¾ cups of egg whites
- 2 teaspoons of pure vanilla
- ½ teaspoon of salt

- 3 cups of butter, soft
- 1 cup of dulce de leche

Instructions:

In a pot set over medium warmness, upload withinside the white sugar. Cover with water. Allow coming to a boil. Cook for a couple of minutes or till it reaches a temperature of 238 degrees.

In a separate bowl, upload withinside the egg whites. Beat with an electric powered mixer till

peaks begin to form.

Add withinside the warm sugar blend. Continue to overcome for 20 mins or

till cooled. Slowly upload withinside the butter pieces. Continue to combine

till fluffy consistency.

Add withinside the sprint of salt, natural vanilla, and dulce de leche. Continue to overcome till incorporated.

 Serve immediately.

19. Peanut Butter Buttercream

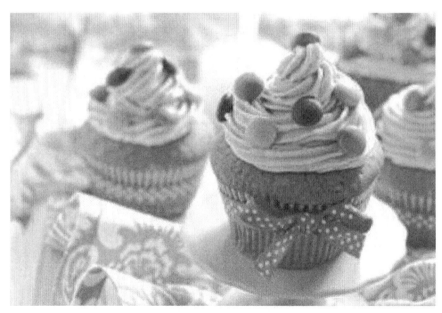

This is one in all my all-time favored buttercream recipes and after you get a flavor of it, I comprehend it becomes one in all your favorites as nicely.

Serving Size: 4 servings

Cooking Time: 5 minutes

Ingredients:

- 1 cup of creamy peanut butter
- 2 sticks of butter, soft
- 4 cups of powdered sugar
- ¼ cup + 2 tablespoons of whole milk
- 2 teaspoons of pure vanilla
- Dash of salt

Instructions:

In the bowl of a stand mixer, upload withinside the butter. Beat on the best placing for two mins or till easy consistency.

Add withinside the creamy peanut butter. Continue to overcome till lightly blended.

Add withinside the powdered sugar, complete milk, and natural vanilla. Continue to overcome for three to five mins or till fluffy consistency.

Add withinside the sprint of salt. Continue to overcome till incorporated. Use immediately.

20. Cake Batter Buttercream Frosting

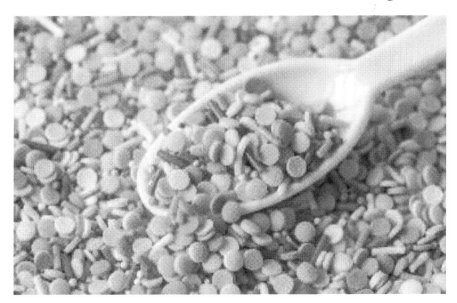

Make this scrumptious buttercream frosting in your subsequent birthday deal with which you are preparing. Made with cake blend and sprinkles, this tasty buttercream frosting becomes everyone's favored frosting.

Serving Size: 4 servings

Cooking Time: 10 minutes

Ingredients:

- 4 cups of powdered sugar
- 1 cup of butter
- 1 cup of cake mix
- 1 teaspoon of pure vanilla
- ¼ cup of whole milk
- ¼ cup of rainbow sprinkles

Instructions:

In a bowl, upload withinside the powdered sugar and cake blend. Stir nicely to combine.

Add withinside the butter and natural vanilla. Beat with an electric powered mixer till mixed.

Add withinside the complete milk. Continue to overcome for two to a few mins or till fluffy consistency.

Add withinside the rainbow sprinkles. Fold lightly to incorporate. Use immediately.

21. White Chocolate Buttercream

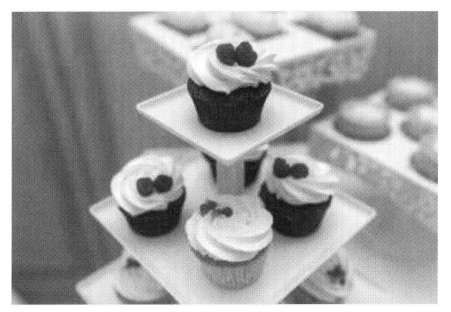

This scrumptious buttercream frosting is straightforward to make and it's miles ideal to pipe onto macarons and unique desserts for the ones unique occasions.

Serving Size: 12 servings

Cooking Time: 10 minutes

Ingredients:

- 1 cup of butter
- 1 cup of powdered sugar
- ¾ cup of white chocolate, broken into pieces
- Whole milk, as needed

Instructions:

In a bowl set over a saucepan packed with simmering water, upload withinside the white chocolate pieces. Allow cooking for two to a few mins or till melted. Remove and set aside.

In a separate bowl, upload withinside the butter. Beat with an electric powered mixer for two to a few

mins or till easy consistency.

Add withinside the powdered sugar. Continue to overcome till fluffy consistency. Add withinside the melted white chocolate. Beat till lightly incorporated.

Use immediately.

22. Margarita Buttercream

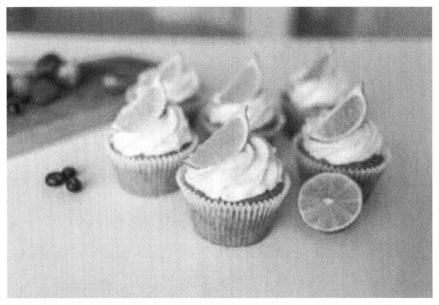

This buttercream frosting tastes similar to a delectable margarita, however it's miles even sweeter and two times as scrumptious. It is straightforward to make, you may need to make it as frequently as possible.

Serving Size: 36 servings

Cooking Time: 25 minutes

Ingredients:

- 6 cups of white sugar
- 1 ¾ cups of egg whites
- 2 teaspoons of pure vanilla
- ½ teaspoon of salt
- 3 cups of butter, soft
- 1 teaspoon of lemon zest
- 1 teaspoon of lime zest
- 1/8 cup of tequila

Instructions:

In a pot set over medium heat, upload withinside the white sugar. Cover with water. Allow coming to a boil. Cook for a couple of minutes or till it reaches a temperature of 238 degrees.

In a separate bowl, upload withinside the egg whites. Beat with an electric powered mixer till peaks start to form.

Add withinside the warm sugar blend. Continue to overcome for 20 mins or till cooled. Slowly upload withinside the butter pieces. Continue to combine till fluffy consistency.

Add withinside the sprint of salt, natural vanilla, lemon zest, lime zest and tequila. Continue to overcome till incorporated.

Serve immediately.

23. Salted Caramel Buttercream Frosting

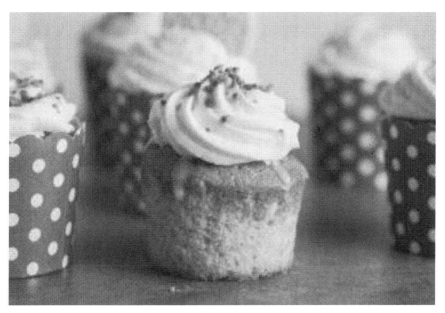

This is a superbly nicely-balanced frosting this is richer than maximum buttercream frostings that you could make today!

Serving Size: 4 servings

Cooking Time: 10 minutes

Ingredients:

- 2 cups of butter

- 1, 14-ounce can of dulce de leche
- 1 teaspoon of pure vanilla
- ½ teaspoon of salt
- 2 to 3 cups of powdered sugar

Instructions:

In a bowl, upload the butter. Beat with an electric powered mixer for five mins or till fluffy consistency.

Add withinside the dulce de leche, natural vanilla, and a sprint of salt. Continue to overcome

till easy consistency.

Add withinside the powdered sugar. Beat on the best placing for two to a few mins or till fluffy consistency.

Use immediately.

24. Simple Vanilla Buttercream Frosting

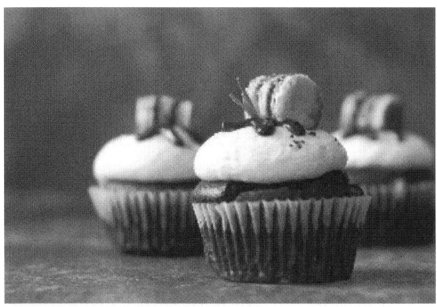

This is one of the creamiest and decadent buttercream frostings that you could make. It is ideal to apply for piping the maximum elaborate designs in your desserts.

Serving Size: 3 servings

Cooking Time: 10 minutes

Ingredients:

- 1 cup of butter, soft
- 4 to 5 cups of powdered sugar
- ¼ cup of heavy whipping cream
- 2 teaspoons of pure vanilla
- Dash of salt

Instructions:

In a bowl, upload the butter. Beat for two mins with an electric powered mixer till creamy consistency.

Add withinside the powdered sugar, heavy whipping cream and natural vanilla.

Continue to overcome for three mins on the bottom placing. Increase the rate of the electrical mixer to high. Continue to overcome for a further minute or till fluffy consistency.

Add in a sprint of salt. Continue to overcome till incorporated. Use immediately.

25. Oreo Buttercream Frosting

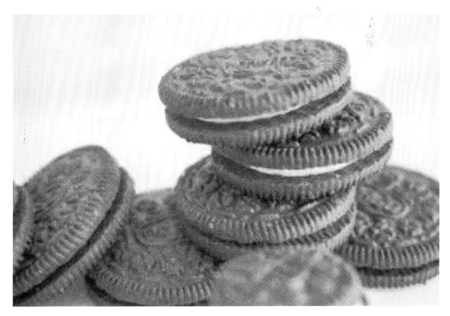

This is the precise frosting to make for the ones choosy eaters on your household. It is ideal to make each time you need to wreck them with some thing unique.

Serving Size: 4 servings

Cooking Time: 10 minutes

Ingredients:

- 10 Oreo cookies
- 1 cup of butter, soft
- 3 cups of powdered sugar
- 1 teaspoon of pure vanilla
- 2 tablespoons of heavy whipping cream

Instructions:

In a meals processor, upload withinside the Oreo cookies. Blend on the best placing till first-rate consistency. Set aside.

In a bowl, upload withinside the butter and powdered sugar. Beat with an electric powered mixer till lightly blended.

Add withinside the natural vanilla and whipping cream. Continue to overcome till easy consistency.

Add withinside the Oreo cookie powder. Continue to overcome till incorporated. Use immediately.

26. Brown Sugar Buttercream Frosting

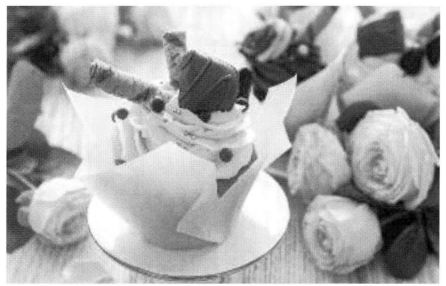

This is a completely unique and high-quality tasting buttercream frosting this is definitely delicious. It is creamy and wealthy in flavor, I recognize you'll like to apply it as regularly as possible.

Serving Size: 4 servings

Cooking Time: 10 minutes

Ingredients:

- 1 cup of butter, soft
- ½ cup of light brown sugar
- 4 cups of powdered sugar
- 2 teaspoons of pure vanilla
- Whole milk, as needed

Instructions:

In a bowl, upload withinside the butter and mild brown sugar. Beat with an electric powered mixer for two mins or till creamy consistency.

Add withinside the natural vanilla. Continue to overcome till mixed.

Add withinside the powdered sugar. Continue to overcome till mixed.

Slowly upload withinside the milk one tablespoon at a time at the same time as beating with the mix. Continue to overcome till the frosting is creamy consistency.

Use immediately.

27. Strawberry Cream Cheese Frosting

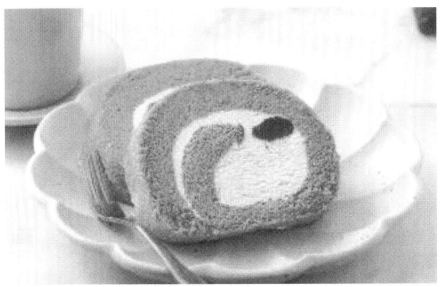

Good buttercream for lots sorts of cakes, consisting of chocolate or white cakes

Serving Size: 4 servings

Cooking Time: 10 minutes

Ingredients:

- 4 ounces Cream cheese, softened
- 4 ounces Butter, unsalted, softened
- 1 1/4 cups Sugar, powdered
- 1/2 cup Cream, heavy whipping
- 1/4 cup Strawberry, puree
- 1/2 teaspoon Vanilla, pure extract

Instructions

Place butter and cream cheese on a kitchen countertop and go away it till it reaches room temperature.

Chill a massive glass or a metallic bowl and the beaters withinside the freezer for 30

mins.

In a relaxing bowl of a stand mixer, upload heavy whipping cream. Beat it on medium pace for five-6 mins till stiff peaks begin to form.

In a separate bowl, beat cream cheese for 1-2 mins till it turns into creamy.

Add softened butter and preserve beating on medium pace for three-four mins till it turns into nicely mixed and easy.

Add strawberry puree and vanilla extract. Beat for any other 2-three mins. Add powdered sugar and beat for four-five mins till it's miles tender and fluffy.

Fold withinside the whipped cream into the cream cheese combination till whipped cream is lightly integrated.

Place into the refrigerator to cool. Store it withinside the fridge for up to 1 week. Beat it with a mixer earlier than the use of it for piping or readorning cakes.

28. Hazelnut Buttercream

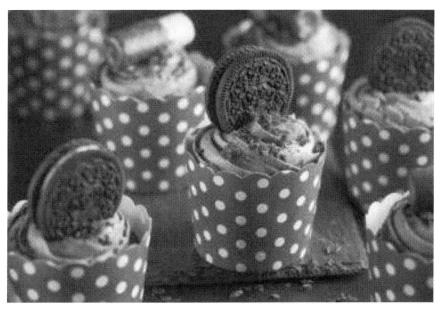

This frosting is super for chocolate cakes.

Serving Size: 4 servings

Cooking Time: 10 minutes

Ingredients:

- 8 ounces Cream cheese, softened

- 4 ounces cup Butter, unsalted, softened
- 1 cup Chocolate-hazelnut, spread
- 1 tablespoon Milk

Instructions

Place butter and cream cheese on a kitchen countertop and go away it till it reaches room temperature.

Beat cream cheese on medium pace in a bowl of a stand mixer outfitted with the paddle attachment for four-five mins till it turns into tender and fluffy.

Little with the aid of using little, upload softened butter and beat on medium pace till all is

integrated and fluffy.

Add hazelnut unfold and milk and preserve beating till easy and fluffy.

Place into the refrigerator to cool. Store it withinside the fridge for up to 1 week. Beat it with a mixer earlier than the use of it for piping or readorning cakes.

29. Amaretto-Maple Cream Cheese Buttercream

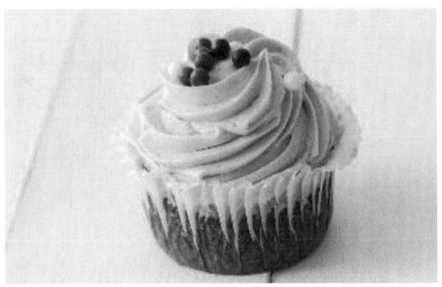

Good buttercream for lots sorts of cakes, consisting of, chocolate cakes

Serving Size: 4 servings

Cooking Time: 10 minutes

Ingredients:

- 8 ounces cream cheese, softened
- 4 ounces Butter, unsalted, softened
- 2 ½ cups Sugar, powdered
- 1/4 cup Amaretto liqueur
- 1 tablespoon Maple syrup, pure
- 1/2 teaspoon Vanilla, pure, extract

Instructions

Place butter and cream cheese on a kitchen countertop and go away it till it reaches room temperature.

In a bowl of stand mixer outfitted with the paddle attachment, beat cream cheese

on medium pace for five-7 mins till it turns into tender and fluffy.

Little with the aid of using little, upload softened butter and beat on medium pace till all is integrated and fluffy.

Add powdered sugar, amaretto liqueur, maple syrup, and vanilla extract. Beat it for any other 1-2 mins till easy and fluffy.

Place into the refrigerator to cool. Store it withinside the fridge for up to 1 week. Beat it with a mixer earlier than the use of it for piping or readorning cakes.

30. Chocolate Marshmallow Fondant

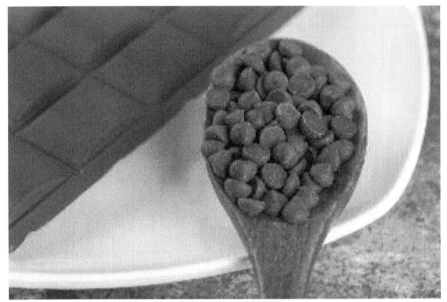

Very true chocolate fondant to cowl chocolate cakes

Serving Size: 4 servings

Cooking Time: 10 minutes

Ingredients:

- 16 ounces Marshmallows, miniature
- 4 cups Sugar, powdered
- 1/2 cup Chocolate chips, dark, bakers
- 2 tablespoons Maple syrup
- 1 teaspoon Coffee, extract

Instructions

In a small bowl, soften marshmallows and continuously stirring on a water bath. Add maple syrup and coffee-flavored extract.

In a small bowl, soften chocolate chips and continuously stirring on a water bath.

Fold withinside the chocolate combination into the marshmallow combination.

Add powdered sugar, one cup at a time, to the chocolate-marshmallow combination, till the dough has a thick, stringy form.

Add a few powdered sugar on a flat operating surface; flip the dough out.

Then, knead till easy and now no longer sticky.

Wrap tightly in a plastic wrap. Let the fondant relaxation from round 8 hours to in a single day at room temperature.

Store withinside the fridge for up to 1 week.

31. Snow White Buttercream

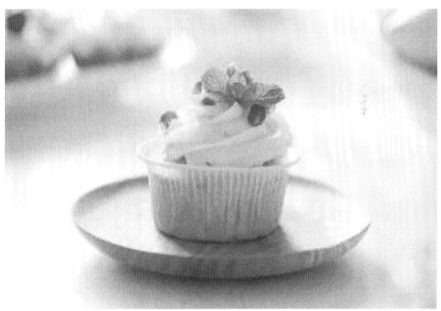

This easy buttercream is right for any form of cupcake or cake.

Serving Size: 4 servings

Cooking Time: 10 minutes

Ingredients

- 1 cup Sugar, cane, powdered
- 1/2 cup Butter, unsalted, softened
- 1/2 cup Shortening, vegetable
- 1/4 cup Flour, all-purpose
- 1 cup Milk
- 1 teaspoon Vanilla, pure, extract

Instructions

In a small saucepan, integrate milk and flour. Cook over medium-excessive warmness till the combination is boiling. Remove from warmness and set apart to cool.

Beat softened butter on medium pace in a bowl of a stand mixer outfitted with the paddle attachment for three-four mins till it turns into tender and fluffy. Then, slowly upload powdered sugar and beat on gradual pace till all is absolutely integrated.

Add vegetable shortening and vanilla. Beat on medium pace for one minute.

Transfer the cooled combination into the bowl with buttercream. Beat it at medium pace till all is absolutely integrated.

Place into the refrigerator to cool. Store it withinside the fridge for up to at least one week. Beat it with a mixer earlier than the use of it for piping or readorning desserts.

32. Christmas Eggnog Buttercream

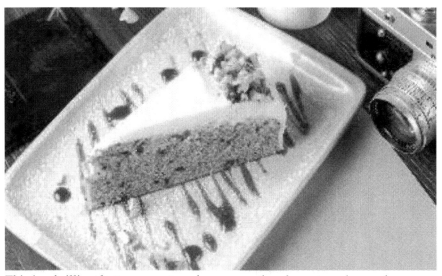

This is a brilliant buttercream to enhance vacation desserts and cupcakes.

Serving Size: 4 servings

Cooking Time: 10 minutes

Ingredients

- 4 cups Sugar, powdered
- 4 ounces Butter, unsalted, softened
- 6 tablespoons Eggnog
- 1 teaspoon Vanilla, pure, extract

Instructions

Place butter on a kitchen countertop and go away it till it reaches room temperature.

In a bowl of a stand mixer, outfitted with the paddle attachment, beat butter on medium velocity for 3-four mins till it will become gentle and light.

Add eggnog and vanilla extract. Beat on medium velocity till all is nicely combined.

Slowly upload powdered sugar. Keep beating till the combination will become gentle and fluffy.

Place into the refrigerator to cool. Store it withinside the fridge for up to at least one week. Beat it with a mixer earlier than the use of it for piping or readorning desserts.

33. Raspberry Buttercream

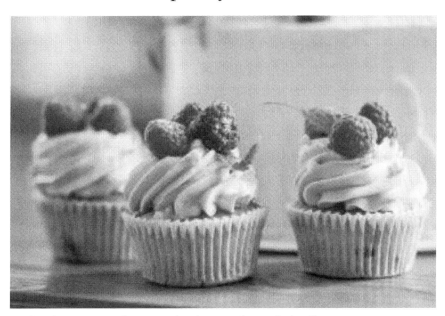

Perfect buttercream for any cake that requires a fruity flavor

Serving Size: 4 servings

Cooking Time: 10 minutes

Ingredients:

For the Buttercream:

- 2 cups Sugar, powdered
- 1 cup Butter, unsalted, softened
- 1 teaspoon Vanilla, pure, extract

For the Raspberry Puree:

- 1 cup Raspberries, fresh or frozen, thawed
- 2 tablespoons Cream, heavy, whipping

Instructions

Make the Puree:

In a blender, puree raspberries and heavy cream till smooth.

Transfer right into a small saucepan, upload tablespoons of powdered sugar, and decrease the liquid through simmering over low heat. Set apart to cool.

Make the Buttercream:

Place butter and on a kitchen countertop and go away it till it reaches room temperature.

In a bowl of a stand mixer, outfitted with the paddle attachment, beat butter on medium velocity for 3-four mins till it will become gentle and light.

Gradually upload powdered sugar and beat till absolutely incorporated. Add vanilla extract and beat once more for 30 seconds.

Add raspberry puree and beat for every other forty five seconds. Do now no longer overbeat.

Place into the refrigerator to cool. Store it withinside the fridge for up to at least one week. Beat it with a mixer earlier than the use of it for piping or readorning desserts.

34. Black Volcano Buttercream

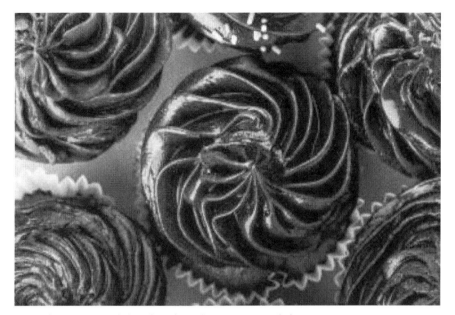

Great buttercream icing for chocolate or caramel desserts

Serving Size: 4 servings

Cooking Time: 10 minutes

Ingredients

- 12 ounces Condensed milk, sweetened
- 8 ounces Butter, unsalted, softened
- 2 cups Sugar, powdered
- 1/2 cup Cocoa powder, Dutch, unsweetened
- 1 teaspoon Vanilla, pure, extract

Instructions

Place butter and on a kitchen countertop and go away it till it reaches room temperature.

In a bowl of a stand mixer, outfitted with the paddle attachment, beat butter on medium velocity for 3-four mins till it will become gentle and light.

Gradually upload powdered sugar and beat till absolutely incorporated. Add vanilla extract and beat once more for 30 seconds.

Add condensed milk and cocoa powder and beat till smooth. Do now no longer overbeat.

Place into the refrigerator to cool. Store it withinside the fridge for up to at least one week. Beat it with a mixer earlier than the use of it for piping or readorning desserts.

35. Avocado Buttercream

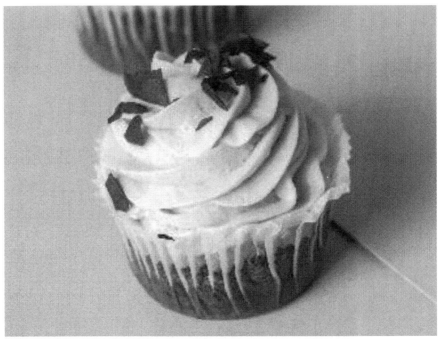

This is a lighter model of buttercream. Great for carrot cupcakes.

Serving Size: 4 servings

Cooking Time: 10 minutes

Ingredients

- 2 cups Sugar, powdered
- 8 ounces Avocado, meat of (approx. 2 avocados)
- 2 teaspoons Lemon juice, freshly squeezed
- 1/2 teaspoon Lemon, extract

Instructions

Peel and pit the avocados. Place avocado meat right into a bowl of a stand mixer, upload lemon juice, and beat for two to a few mins till it lightens in color.

Add powdered sugar (a touch at a time) and beat till smooth. Add the lemon extract and beat for every other 30 seconds to combine.

Place into the refrigerator to cool. Store withinside the fridge for up to one week. Beat it with a mixer earlier than the use of it.

Printed in Great Britain
by Amazon